GIANT CELL ARTHRITIS

UNDERSTANDING THE RISK ELEMENTS FOR GIANT CELL ARTHRITIS

DR. KATE .P

Contents

CHAPTER ONE

INTRODUCTION

An inflammation of the artery lining, which lines the blood channels that supply oxygen-rich blood from your heart to the rest of your body, is known as giant cell arteritis. It usually affects your head's arteries, particularly the ones in your temples. Because of this, giant cell arteritis is sometimes known as cranial arteritis or temporal arteritis.

Headaches, jaw pain, and double or blurry vision are common symptoms of giant cell arteritis. The most dangerous side effects of giant cell arteritis are blindness and, less frequently, stroke.

Giant cell arteritis must be treated quickly to avoid irreversible tissue damage and visual loss. Corticosteroid drugs may avoid visual loss and typically alleviate giant cell arteritis symptoms. It is likely that you will feel better a few days after commencing treatment.

Symptoms

Giant cell arteritis is most commonly characterized by intense headache pain and soreness that typically affects both temples. On the other hand, some persons only have discomfort in one temple or in the front of their head.

Giant cell arthritis symptoms and signs can differ. Some people have what seems like the flu when the condition first starts, including headaches, fever, weariness, and myalgia, or stiffness and aches in the muscles surrounding the shoulders and hips.

The following are typical giant cell arteritis indications and symptoms:

strong, ongoing headache discomfort and tenderness, commonly in the temple region

loss of vision or double vision

Tenderness in the scalp – comb your hair or merely rest your head on a pillow may cause pain, particularly in areas where the arteries are inflamed.

Jaw claudication, or pain in the jaw when you eat or open your mouth wide abrupt, irreversible loss of one eye's eyesight

High temperature

Unexpected weight reduction

Polymyalgia rheumatica is a similar illness that commonly manifests as pain and stiffness in the neck, shoulders, or hips. Polymyalgia rheumatica affects around half of patients with giant cell arteritis.

When to visit a physician

See your doctor right away if you experience any of the following symptoms or if you get a new, persistent headache. Getting treatment as soon as possible after being identified with giant cell arteritis can typically help prevent blindness.

Your arteries are flexible tubes with walls that are thick and elastic. The aorta, the major artery in your body, is where oxygenated blood exits your heart. Following its division into smaller arteries, the aorta supplies blood to every area of your body, including your internal organs and brain.

Some of these arteries enlarge as a result of inflammation brought on by giant cell arteritis, which can occasionally reduce blood flow. It is unclear exactly what triggers the inflammation of these arteries.

Swelling most commonly affects the temporal arteries in your head, which run from immediately in front of your ears up into your scalp, however practically any large or medium-sized artery can be impacted. Sometimes the enlargement just affects a portion of an artery, leaving normal arterial segments intact in between.

RISK ELEMENTS

While the precise etiology of giant cell arteritis remains unknown, a number of variables can raise your risk, such as:

Years old. Almost exclusively affecting older folks, giant cell arteritis rarely strikes those under 50 years old. The average age at commencement of the disease is 70.

Sexual. Giant cell arteritis is roughly twice as common in women.

origins in Northern Europe, particularly Scandinavia. Giant cell arteritis can strike anyone, but it seems to strike more frequently in those born in Northern European nations. Scandinavian-born individuals are especially vulnerable.

rheumatic polymyalgia. Individuals suffering from polymyalgia rheumatica have stiffness and pain in their shoulders, hips, and neck. Giant cell arteritis coexists with polymyalgia rheumatica in about 15% of cases.

The following complications may result from giant cell arteritis:

blindness. The gravest consequence of giant cell arteritis is this. Giant cell arteritis causes swelling that narrows blood arteries, which lowers the quantity of blood that reaches your body's tissues and, consequently, oxygen and essential nutrients. Reduced blood supply to the eyes can result in an abrupt, painless loss of vision in one or, in rare circumstances, both of the eyes. Sadly, blindness is typically irreversible.

Aneurism in the aorta. Aneurysm risk is increased by giant cell arteritis. A weak blood vessel, generally the aorta, the big artery that runs through the middle of your chest and abdomen, can expand and become an aneurysm. Because it has the potential to rupture and cause potentially fatal internal bleeding, an aortic aneurysm is a dangerous condition. Your doctor may use yearly chest X-rays or other imaging tests, like an MRI, CT scan, or ultrasound, to check on the condition of your aorta because it can happen years after giant cell arteritis was first diagnosed.

a stroke. A blood clot may occasionally form in an artery that is compromised, completely blocking blood flow, depriving a portion of your brain of vital oxygen and nutrients, and potentially leading to a stroke. This is an unusual but significant side effect of giant cell arteritis.

Getting Ready for Your Consultation

The first place you should probably go if you suspect giant cell arteritis is your primary care physician. In certain situations, your physician might also recommend that you see an ophthalmologist (specialist in eyes), a neurologist (specialist in the brain and neurological system) if you're experiencing headaches, or a rheumatologist (specialist in joints) if you're experiencing symptoms of polymyalgia rheumatica.

It's a good idea to be prepared because meetings can run short and there might be a lot to talk about. Here are some tips to help you prepare and know what to anticipate from your physician.

What you're capable of

Read any restrictions about appointments in advance. Make sure to inquire about any prior requirements when scheduling the appointment. Prior to the consultation, you might need to follow specific guidelines for some tests used to diagnose giant cell arteritis.

Jot down any symptoms you're having, even if they don't seem to be connected to the reason you made the visit.

CHAPTER TWO

Important personal details, such as significant stressors or recent life transitions, should be included.

List all of the vitamins, minerals, and prescription drugs you now take, along with the dosage details.

Bring a friend or family member with you. It might occasionally be challenging to recall everything that was said to you during an appointment. It's possible that someone with you will recall something you overlooked or forgot.

Prepare a list of inquiries for your physician

Making the most of your time with your doctor and maybe making sure you cover all the topics that are important to you can be accomplished by preparing a list of questions in advance. Some fundamental inquiries for your physician regarding giant cell arteritis are as follows:

Which of my symptoms is most likely to be the cause?

Exist any more potential reasons?

Which tests are necessary to verify the diagnosis? Do you need to prepare in any way for these tests?

What alternatives do I have for treatment?

What kinds of adverse drug reactions might I anticipate?

What is the duration of my pharmaceutical regimen and what is the outlook for the future?

Is giant cell arteritis going to reappear?

These additional medical conditions affect me. How can I and my partner best manage these conditions?

Do I need to make any dietary changes? Do I require any supplements to be taken?

Are there any printed materials, such as brochures, that I can bring with me? Which websites would you suggest?

Do not be afraid to ask any more questions that come up during your session, in addition to the ones you have prepared for your doctor.

What to anticipate from your physician

You'll probably be asked a lot of questions by your doctor. Being prepared to respond to them could buy you extra time to discuss topics you'd like to take more time to cover. Your physician might inquire:

When did you start feeling the effects?

Have you experienced constant symptoms or just sporadic ones?

What level of severity do you have?

What appears to alleviate your problems, if anything?

What seems to exacerbate your symptoms, if anything?

What you can accomplish in the interim

Consult your physician about if taking acetaminophen (Tylenol, etc.), ibuprofen (Advil, Motrin IB, etc.), or naproxen (Aleve) can help reduce headache pain or soreness.

Exams and diagnosis

Because of how many common ailments its early symptoms mirror, giant cell arteritis can be challenging to diagnose. Your doctor will therefore make an effort to rule out any more potential reasons of your issue.

You might undergo some or all of the following tests to aid in the diagnosis of giant cell arteritis:

physical examination. Your doctor will probably ask you about your symptoms and medical history in addition to doing a full physical examination and focusing especially on your temporal arteries. One or both of these arteries are frequently painful, have a weaker pulse, and feel and look like hard cords.

blood examinations. Your doctor may order a blood test to measure your erythrocyte sedimentation rate, sometimes known as the "sed rate," if they think you have giant cell arteritis.

This test calculates the rate at which red blood cells settle to the bottom of a blood tube. Rapidly declining red blood cells could be a sign of inflammation in your body.

Additionally, a test measuring C-reactive protein (CRP), which your liver generates when inflammation is present, can be performed on you. You may monitor your progress during treatment with the same tests.

autopsy. The most reliable method of verifying a giant cell arteritis diagnosis is to obtain a biopsy, or little sample, from the temporal artery. It could be necessary to take more than one sample because the inflammation could not affect the entire artery. Under local anesthetic, the surgery is carried done as an outpatient with minimal discomfort and scarring typically. In a lab, the sample is inspected under a microscope.

The artery will frequently exhibit inflammation containing abnormally big cells, known as giant cells, which are responsible for the disease's name if you have giant cell arteritis. Sadly, a biopsy is not infallible. Giant cell arteritis can occur in spite of a negative biopsy result. Your doctor might suggest getting another temporal artery biopsy on the other side of your head if the results are unclear.

Imaging studies can be used to both diagnose giant cell arteritis and track the course of treatment, while a temporal artery biopsy remains the standard diagnostic for this condition. Potential examinations consist of:

MRA stands for magnetic resonance imaging. This test creates fine-grained images of your blood arteries by combining the use of magnetic resonance imaging (MRI) and a contrast agent. Because the test is done in a tube-shaped equipment, let your doctor know in advance if you feel uncomfortable being confined in a small space.

Ultrasound Doppler. This test creates images of your blood flowing through your blood vessels using sound waves.

PET, or Positron Emission Tomography. Through the use of an intravenous tracer solution containing a small quantity of radioactive material, a PET scan can identify areas of inflammation and provide detailed images of your blood arteries.

MEDICATIONS AND SUBTLES

Prednisone is one corticosteroid medication used in high dosages to treat giant cell arteritis. Your doctor will probably start medication even before doing a biopsy to confirm the diagnosis because vision loss must be prevented immediately.

Within a few days, you should feel better, but you might need to keep taking the drug for up to two years. Your doctor may start reducing the dosage after the first month until you reach the lowest level of corticosteroids required to reduce inflammation, as determined by sedation rate and

CRP testing. It's possible that some of your symptoms will come back during this taper.

How do corticosteroids work?

Strong anti-inflammatory medications called corticosteroids work by simulating the actions of hormones secreted by your adrenal glands. Although long-term use of the medications, particularly at high doses, can result in a number of dangerous side effects, the pharmaceuticals can successfully reduce pain.

Due to their increased susceptibility to illnesses that may potentially be brought on by corticosteroids, older persons, who are the group most likely to receive treatment for giant cell arteritis, are especially vulnerable to adverse effects. Among them are:

The osteoporosis

elevated blood pressure

weakened muscles

glaucoma

The cataracts

The following are additional adverse effects of corticosteroid therapy:

Gaining weight

elevated blood sugar levels, which can occasionally result in diabetes

Thin skin and more frequent bruises

weakened immune system, which increases the risk of infection and slows the healing process

Your doctor will likely evaluate your bone density and may prescribe calcium and vitamin D supplements or other medications to assist prevent bone loss in order to counteract the probable negative effects of corticosteroid treatment. In order to maintain blood pressure within a normal range, your doctor may additionally monitor your blood pressure and prescribe medication, food modifications, and exercise regimen. When the corticosteroid treatment is stopped, the majority of side effects disappear.

Consult your physician about starting anti-platelet medication (81–100 mg of aspirin each day). When taken regularly, aspirin can lower the risk of stroke and blindness.

WAY OF LIFE AND DOMESTIC MEDICINE

The prognosis for giant cell arteritis is typically very good if it is identified and treated quickly. When you start corticosteroid treatment, your symptoms should go away immediately, and you shouldn't have any visual effects. Managing any drug side effects can be your biggest obstacle in this situation. The ideas listed below could be beneficial:

Consume a balanced diet. Eating a healthy diet can help stave off conditions like diabetes, high blood pressure, and thinning bones. Limit your intake of salt, sweets, and alcohol and place an emphasis on nutritious grains, lean meats, and fish. Make sure you are getting enough calcium and vitamin D. Experts advise consuming 800 international units (IU) of vitamin D and 1,000–1,200 mg of calcium daily. To determine the appropriate dosage for you, consult your physician.

Engage in regular exercise. Walking is a good type of aerobic exercise that can help avoid diabetes, high blood pressure, and bone loss. It is also good for your lungs and heart. Furthermore, a lot of people discover that exercising enhances their general sense of wellbeing and mood. If you're not accustomed to working out, begin slowly and increase your time gradually. Try to work out for at least half an hour most days. You can create a personalized workout regimen with the assistance of your physician.

Adapting and providing assistance

Acquiring comprehensive knowledge about giant cell arteritis and its management might enhance your sense of control over your illness. You can ask questions of your healthcare staff, and you can also get assistance from online support groups. Be aware of any potential negative effects from any medications you take, and let your doctor know if anything changes with your health.

THE END